HOW TO BECOME SMILE EVERYDAY
The antidotes of sadness and failure.

By

Taylor Francis

Disclaimer

Table of Content

"Happiness is life. Try it your life will never remain the same "

INTRODUCTION

Whether it's a trip, a ceremony, or a marriage, sometimes we create grand plans that are supposed to bring enjoyment into our lives. But we can rely on the little things in life to make us happy forever. When we enjoy and appreciate the little things, our thankfulness

will spread to other spheres as well. Here are a few straightforward joys that merit making an effort to enjoy often.

Recently cut grass

Every aspect of enjoying freshly cut grass. It is invigorating to the senses and has a fresh scent and sensation beneath your bare feet.
As long as the weather permits it, try to do this a few times a year at the very least.

Smiles Exchanged and Received

What better approach is to enjoy a basic pleasure for nothing? Don't only smile at your pals; also smile at strangers

you pass on the street. You won't believe how nice it feels to first see other people's amazement, followed by their grins in response.

The After-Workout Endorphin Rush

You will get an endorphin surge as a reward for exerting yourself throughout a challenging workout. Your day will become better thanks to these healthy, happy chemicals. Exercise in the morning to take advantage of the endorphin high and be more effective for the rest of the day.

Your Favorite Food Enjoyed

Allow yourself to sometimes indulge in your favorite meal, even if it's not the healthiest option. Your feelings about your favorite cuisine will provide you with a little boost of joy. Use this strategy to make your favorite meal taste even better than normal since studies have shown that if you skip a specific cuisine for some time, it will be significantly more delightful the next time you consume it.

Tea or Coffee in a Hot Cup

Some of us can get by on our daily cup of coffee or tea. It may be enjoyable even if it becomes a routine. Spend some peaceful time indulging in your beverage of choice as you drink.

developing snow angels

Not only for children, though. Put on some warm clothing, then plunge yourself into the snow. Simply embrace the sense of pure joy that building snow angels may provide; feeling stupid about it won't harm the experience.

Until It Hurts, Laughing

Laughter is a healing force. Everyone should have the chance to laugh so hard they cry at least once a day. Spend some time laughing to relieve your tension, whether it be with a funny buddy or a fantastic movie.

Having a massage

Try a massage if you've never experienced one. Your worries will seem as if they are dissipating during this hour of complete relaxation. Even more people have access to massages because of work perks.

Taking a Rainy Walk

One of life's wonderful, simple joys is strolling in the rain. Go outdoors, dressed warmly, with or without an umbrella. As you walk through the rain, let it spray over your face. For nostalgia's sake, jump in at least one puddle.

Although difficult to find, expensive enjoyment is fantastic. Spend some time enjoying one of these simple pleasures instead of waiting for your next trip. You will experience daily happiness if you can learn to appreciate the little things that are there in front of you.

Chapter 1

Is money necessary for happiness?

As they say, "Money can't buy you happiness." But can it? While having enough money might help reduce stress, having too much of it won't make you happier than anybody else. So, can you purchase pleasure with money or not? Here are some ideas to consider on the matter.

You Can Only Get So Much Happiness for Your Money

According to studies, being able to provide for your family's needs and your own brings satisfaction. In general, poor persons are less content than those whose needs are satisfied. It would be easier for you to be content if you could pay your expenses and have enough money to get by.

Money in Excess Doesn't Equal Happiness in Excess

But having more money than you need won't make you happier. Happiness and wealth are not inversely related. A person who has enough money to purchase a big home and plenty of automobiles may not necessarily be happier than someone who just has what they need.

Money Has Its Stresses

When you have money, you have tension. No matter how much or little you have, you're probably aware of this tension. In addition to the anxiety that comes with knowing that you must use your

resources properly, being affluent attracts those who have bad intentions.

What Leaves Is More Important Than What Enters

Your happiness is more dependent on what you spend your money on and where it goes after you take it than on how much you earn. You might feel more content by following certain financial guidelines. Depending on where and to whom you give your money, you may or may not have benefited from possessing it.

Spend money on memories rather than things.

It's not proven that buying more stuff would make someone happier. Although buying durable goods can seem like a smart choice, research has shown that we often adapt to what we get. These possessions do not continue to offer unending bliss.

When money is spent on events that leave us with enduring memories, we are more likely to enjoy long-term happiness. Whether this is taking a solo or family trip or just scheduling occasional pleasant activities...

Make careful to build experiences rather than buying things that will eventually become obsolete.

Toss it out

One of the most fulfilling things you can do with your money is to give. Find a way to give back and share what you have, whether it's for a good cause or a buddy in need. This is a method of spending that will benefit the individual in the long run.

The quick answer is no; having money does not guarantee happiness. But having money may help you avoid stress, which

can make your existing happiness lessened. No matter how much money you have, utilize these suggestions to help you find the degree of happiness you want and have a happy life.

We've all been told not to worry too much about the little things.

One of the largest ways to add needless suffering to one's life is to allow oneself to get stressed up about little matters.
Simply by learning to not allow the small things to bother us, we may prevent many unpleasant emotions and even health issues.
Think of the big picture.

Chapter 2

Don't worry about little things

When something happens that makes you want to scream, weigh its importance for the rest of your life and the world at large. One hour before your visitors are scheduled to arrive, you could have spilled your cake mix on the floor. If you don't have a freshly made cake for your pals, would they still adore you and have a good time? If so, maybe you need to direct your focus elsewhere

instead of berating yourself for this little error.

Keep in Mind That Everyone Makes Mistakes

Consider the reality that everyone makes errors when a little issue threatens to derail your view and mood. Remember that errors are a common aspect of life and happen to everyone, whether you or someone else is to blame for the scenario that seems like a train catastrophe. Don't let one poor experience catch you off guard.

Let Others Go

When you believe that another person has caused you more effort or worry, it might be difficult to forgive them. You may be tempted to yell at someone when they hit the back of your car.

However, pause for a moment and consider how you may feel if you were in their shoes. Choose empathy instead of acting and feeling as if you've never made a mistake.

Accept Yourself

Compared to forgiving ourselves, forgiving others might be a

straightforward process. There are numerous times when we

treat ourselves more cruelly than we ever allow a friend to. If you are having trouble forgiving yourself, consider how you would react if a close friend committed a mistake. Before you bully yourself, take a moment to reflect. If you find it difficult to stop yourself from thinking negatively whenever you fall short of perfection, you may want to consider getting professional assistance.

Consider if it will matter in ten years.

Everybody has difficulties, and most of the time, they all appear quite large. Though perception is not always accurate, it is our responsibility to put things into perspective so that we may effectively handle whatever comes our way.

When something bad occurs in your life, consider if it will still be relevant in 15 years. Let it go if it won't. You may be tempted to lose your cool if someone throws you the middle finger when you're stuck in traffic, but it's just not worth it. Save your feelings for situations that will change your life and need all of your focus.

Two options exist when anything goes wrong. Either let it go or let your temper flare up. You will be grateful for your personal perspective change and the life-changing satisfaction that comes from choosing not to worry about the little things.

Chapter 3

consider now is, are you happy?

A commonality shared by practically everyone is the desire to be happy. However, it is not always simple to find happiness or to assess your level of pleasure once you feel as if you ought to be in a certain frame of mind.

Every life will have highs and lows, thus it is useful to have a yardstick by which to determine whether or not we have attained happiness.

Am I Excited for the Day When I Wake Up?

This gives away your level of inner contentment. Do you sense dread and anxiety when you awaken each morning or do you feel ready to face the day? If you have a bad attitude when you get up every morning, it's hard to be cheerful.

Do I Enjoy My Primary Profession?

There should be excitement when you consider going there, regardless of whether you are

working, going to school, or doing anything else. Your choice to work may not be an option since there are certain things we must do, like pay the rent. However, you do have a choice as to where you work. Change it if you don't like it.

Am I Happy with the People I Spend the Most Time With?

The individuals that you spend the most of your time with will have the biggest impact on you. Likely, you will ultimately turn out to be the same kind of person if you are bitter, demoralizing,

and unmotivated. Find new pals if your current ones are depressing. Spend your spare time with people who will make your life happier and who can help you make lasting memories that will make you happy.

Do I Enjoy Being Me?

The ability to accept and love oneself for who you are is

essential to happiness. If you don't, you must ascertain why. Make the required adjustments, then decide to accept yourself, warts and all.

Do I fear or anticipate the future?

Feeling comfortable and confident about the future is a component of happiness. Even if our times are unpredictable, we don't have to spend every day in terror. Develop your self-assurance little by little, and think about seeking counseling

if you experience more than sporadic concern when you ponder the future.

Do I Know What My Life Is For?

Every person is here for a reason. You are a special gift to the world because of something about you. Your happiness and self-worth will suffer if you have not yet realized this about yourself. There are several quizzes and publications devoted to figuring out your life's purpose. Spend some time

learning more and figuring out what in life gives you the greatest satisfaction.
Happiness is a worthwhile goal. It's critical to understand your wiring as well as what it takes to be content with who you are and where you are in life. You will be well on your way to living a life

of real happiness if you ask yourself these questions and then take some time to reflect on your responses.

Chapter 4

The Relationship Between Happiness and Food

Did you know that eating may have a significant positive or negative impact on your mood? Food has the power to help or hurt you in every aspect of your life, including your happiness.

You may take care of your health and mind and embrace happiness by being knowledgeable about the foods to eat and stay away from.

Foods that Increase Happiness

You want to improve your mood, so why not take advantage of what Mother Nature has to offer? To begin with, search for meals that are abundant in good fats. These fats, including omega-3 fatty acids, are essential to the health of our brains and help our nerve cells communicate more

effectively, which has a positive impact on our happiness and mood. The best foods to eat are walnuts, pumpkin seeds, and fish oil. It has been shown that omega-3 fatty acids are just as

effective in treating depression as generic antidepressants. Berries are yet another fantastic technique to increase happiness. They contain anthocyanin's, which are good for your brain because they help it work. The stress-fighting vitamin C found in oranges, fresh peppers, and kiwis is abundant. Even dark chocolate is recognized as a mood booster, while leafy vegetables increase your folic acid consumption. Dates and bananas are common meals that are known to raise serotonin levels. Dehydration hurts both your mood and your ability to think clearly, so be sure to drink

lots of water to keep well-hydrated.

Foods That Take Your Joy Away

If you want to be happy, you should avoid sugar over all other foods. The sugar high, which is quickly followed by a fall, prepares you for a brief, deceptive rush of energy. Additionally, sugar has been linked to immune system damage and depression.

Coffee is known to cause worry, which also steals happiness. Wheat interferes with the production of serotonin, which

aggravates sadness. Although some people experience brief euphoria after ingesting alcohol, the sensation often becomes negative. Alcohol is associated with moodiness.

Cortisol, the hormone that causes stress, has been proven

to be reduced by vitamin C. It's a good idea to take a daily supplement unless you are receiving a significant quantity of this vitamin through your food. You need to think about taking a supplement since a folic acid deficiency has been connected to melancholy. Additionally useful for a mood boost naturally are omega-3

fatty acids and vitamin B12. Vitamin B complex, Co-Enzyme Q10, and resveratrol are supplements that may help you manage unhealthy appetites. You should make the most of food to the fullest extent possible since it has such a significant impact on your mood. Turn your plate into a potent tool that will battle anxiety and despair and help you create and keep happiness rather than merely picking your meal based on what you are now craving.

You should have the opportunity to experience pleasure, and changing your

eating habits may help you live a happier life. See the difference it makes when you choose your meal based on your mood.

Chapter 5

Seven Affirmations to Make You Happier

There are several methods for raising your level of happiness,

as well as several quick fixes. By telling yourself mantras throughout the day, you will discover that feeling joyful starts to flow effortlessly to you. Our words have power.

Here are seven affirmations that, when used often, may transform your life.

I Am Stunning

You may avoid sinking into a pit of self-hatred by remembering these three words. Too many people disregard their worth and fail to recognize their incredible abilities, unique beauty, and uniqueness. For the words to come to you when you need them the most, repeat this mantra often.

I Appreciate You

A certain path to pleasure is gratitude. Being thankful is making an effort to keep in mind all the blessings in your life. This

optimistic outlook then draws even better things to itself.

I always cherish myself.

Self-love is one of life's most crucial lessons. Repeat these phrases until you feel as if you have reached a complete state of respect and love for yourself. Say them both when you are proud of yourself and when you are upset or dissatisfied with yourself.

I Draw Positive Things for Myself

Believing that wonderful things and favorable circumstances are coming your way will encourage them to do so. You

will pull great things to you if you see yourself as a magnet for anything amazing. You will notice that when you repeat this mantra often, your life will get richer because of your self-assurance and optimistic outlook.

I Pull Healthy Individuals Into My Life

The wrong individuals will prevent us from moving forward, even under ideal

conditions. Make a group of people who share your

optimism and hope for the future. When you find yourself tempted to engage in drama, remind yourself to stay away from it by repeating this mantra to yourself.

I am capable of everything I put my mind to.

Being confident in your abilities and yourself will help you succeed. You will discover limitless enjoyment in knowing that you can do everything you put your mind to. Speak these phrases when you are trying to alter your circumstances and remember that you can do so.

I've Got a Goal

Life will seem worthless and hollow without a sense of purpose, regardless of how much money someone earns or how much they achieve. You may study your life and determine your unique mission using several books that have been published on the topic.

Consider the things you are attracted to and like, as well as what makes you feel the

happiest. This phrase reminds you that you

have something unique to give the world.
Mantras are an excellent approach to put us on the road to happiness since words have a lot of power. You will be happy when you utilize your words to improve the quality of your life. Find out what a difference it will make for you if you repeat these mantras.

Chapter 6

Characteristics and Contentment

It seems that some folks are just more content than others. It's not necessarily restricted to those with simple lifestyles, though. Joyful people seem to possess qualities that others don't.

Personality type is one thing that is for sure. What role does it have in the quest for pleasure for oneself? The following is a list of personality qualities and how

they impact how you feel about yourself.

Perfectionism

In comparison to personality types who are more forgiving of different outcomes, perfectionism tends to make people less pleased about themselves and others. A perfectionist will be satisfied

with a work well done, but their enjoyment will be short-lived because of their constant attention on the next major undertaking. Your happiness will increase if you start to embrace the process rather than

enforcing rigid standards on yourself.

Dreaming

Happy people often have dreams. Despite the tendency that dreamers have to procrastinate, which causes tension, there is always something to dream about again after the stress has gone. We may learn a lot from dreamers as we pursue pleasure in life, even if it is not how we were normally born. You will discover the delight in this simple practice if you consider what you want from life and

spend a little amount of time each day relishing the concept of that particular thing.

Organization

Those with personalities that tend toward organization have

a lot going for them, but even in this case, too much of a good thing may be detrimental. There is a balance between the two. Organizing yourself too much will cause you to overlook the little things that should be appreciated along the road. On the other side, if you are very unorganized, you will

get frustrated when things do not go as you had hoped.
Find a happy medium and decide to structure yourself just enough to improve operations.

Positivity

One personality attribute that positively impacts one's level of happiness daily is positivity. While some individuals naturally exhibit this feature, others must make an effort to avoid it. No matter which side you typically gravitate toward, make decisions that will help you respond positively and increase your confidence in the course of life.

When you allow your energy to change from negative to positive, you'll discover that happiness comes to you naturally.

Existing in the Present

You may choose to live in the present whether you're an extrovert or an introvert. Being present for every stage of the trip is essential to achieving happiness since we only get to experience our lives once.
While some individuals find this simpler, others must put out more effort. Whatever your inclination, decide to act without

reservation and with all of your heart to have no regrets and to have profound delight. Although we can't alter our

characteristics, we may still benefit from one another. An inherent propensity towards or away from happiness exists in people with various personalities and personality features. Utilize the characteristics you have been given and focus all of your attention on leading a happy life.

Chapters 7

Why Being Present in the Moment Increases Happiness

Everyone is aware that dwelling on the past may bring one down, but why? How might life in the future work?

We must strike a balance, but if we want to live happy lives, we must put more of our attention on being present. It has been established that the greatest approach to finding and maintaining happiness is to live in the present. Here's why.

The past is irreversible.

We all have regrets about some aspect of the past, but there is nothing we can do to alter it. We may utilize the energy to improve the circumstances we are in right now rather than spending time and energy mourning over things that are long gone and beyond our power to alter. Move forward after taking what lessons you can from the past.

We can't know what the future will bring.

The future is unpredictable, so don't worry about what it may hold. You can only plan for certain things, and worrying about what the future may bring just adds stress, which may lead to physical and mental health issues. Live in the present and decide to concentrate on it. Make choices focused on what is positive in your life at this very time rather than worrying about the consequences they may have in the future. This will lessen the propensities of anxiety and despair.

It Compels You to Be Here

We tend to lose focus on what is immediately in front of us when we spend more time thinking about the past or the future than the present. Perhaps a job project is taking up all of your time and energy right now. Your current situation may entail little children who need lunch to be set out and who have runny noses.

You will get more out of your life if you truly embrace the moment. You will finally be able to quit destroying your

current happiness out of guilt over previous actions or dread of what could happen ahead.

Be grateful for the people you are seeing right now and the possibilities that are coming your way right now. You won't look back and lament your misguided attention because you will take the sweet recollections of the times you learned to enjoy with you into the future.

A balanced outlook

It's crucial to stay present. It's crucial to maintain a balanced attention. When you consider the future, make the preparations you'll need to take advantage of that period later

since, one day, you'll be living "at the moment" and the future will be that. Planning for the future is important, but you shouldn't allow it to negatively affect your life. You won't experience tension from focusing too much on one thing if you maintain balance.
One of the best things you can do for yourself is to practice present-moment living. When

we decide to appreciate and live in the now rather than longing for the past or the future, we are happier. You will experience genuine pleasure by making the most of the time and the life you have right now.

Chapter 8

Satisfaction and Hormones

Hormones don't usually get a lot of respect. Why are they important for happiness? Since hormones have a big impact on this feeling, we need to know how they work and how we may use this emotion to our advantage.

How Do Hormones Work?

Hormones are distinct chemical messengers that control most

biological processes. The endocrine glands create these distinct signals, which are essential for our body to function properly.
Depending on how we treat our bodies and the things we surround ourselves with, these hormones may help us. By knowing what they do and how

we may be able to support them in doing so, we might be able to get closer to our goal of happiness.

What Hormones Are Related to Happiness?

It has been shown that several hormones boost happiness. The three main ones are dopamine, oxytocin, and serotonin. Serotonin has received a lot of attention lately. It is a neurotransmitter that carries information between various brain regions. Problems may

occur when this hormone is not functioning properly or is present in the body in inadequate amounts, both of which are necessary for preventing depression and other mental diseases.
The "love hormone" oxytocin, among other things, fosters

social competence and lessens fear in people.
Dopamine, another neurotransmitter that is produced in response to pleasurable and unexpected events, is well known for its role

in instructing the brain about rewards.

How to Naturally Balance Your Hormones

A careful balance of hormones is necessary for optimal performance. Both short-term and long-term health consequences may result from having too much or too

little of any hormone. Since our happiness relies on achieving a healthy balance for all of our hormones, it would be wise for us to do our best to accomplish so since it would enable us to foster a happy environment. To keep your hormones functioning properly and in balance, it's important to get enough sleep each night, exercise often, and avoid exposure to pollutants. As much as you can, lessen your level of stress, and if at all possible, avoid using birth control pills.

nutrients and vitamins for hormone balance

Hormones, which are compounds that control several

body processes, Including duplication, metabolism, and stress management, are created by the endocrine system.

Your hormones have an impact on your health and happiness. When you have a hormonal imbalance, which happens when your body generates too much or too little of a certain hormone or is unable to utilize hormones effectively, even little variations

in hormone levels may have big impacts.

Mood swings and irritability, Hot flashes, exhaustion and

poor energy, difficulty sleeping, anxiety, weight increase (particularly belly feeds, decreased libido, and trouble sleeping are common signs of hormone imbalances in women. Breast discomfort and sensitivity. Fog in the head, brittle hair, and dull, dry skin.

How can I control my hormone levels?

Conventional medicine still relies on harmful prescription

synthetic hormones to manage women's hormonal

problems, which is a frustrating Band-Aid fix.

The optimal approaches to treating female hormone imbalances, however, are very different according to natural health. The first stage is identifying the underlying cause of the imbalance, which is followed by effective dietary and lifestyle changes, encouragement of healthy hormone production, and the addition of vitamins, minerals, herbs, and other nutritional supplements that support hormonal balance.

the causes of hormonal imbalances

During a woman's menstrual cycle, perimenopause, postpartum period, and other hormonally active times, hormone imbalances often manifest. When hormone levels fluctuate rapidly throughout key developmental

stages, anything might go wrong more of cause.

Hormonal imbalances may also be brought on by underlying medical problems including PCOS (polycystic ovarian syndrome), endometriosis, adrenal fatigue, or

hypothyroidism (low thyroid). Your body's ability to control your hormones at any one period in your life may be influenced by the foods you eat, how much sleep you get, your exposure to toxins, and how much stress you face in your daily life.

Can vitamins help with hormone regulation?

The endocrine glands need certain micronutrients to operate correctly and create hormones. People with low

thyroid, for example, may lack iodine and selenium, two

minerals required by the thyroid gland to produce and use thyroid hormones. Herbs and other organic substances may be able to help with hormone imbalances via therapeutic means. Ashwagandha is a traditional remedy and a part of our Herbal Equilibrium And adaptation formulas. It is an adaptogenic herb known for its ability to re-regulate excessive cortisol, an adrenal imbalance related to chronic stress and anxiety. If you experience the

hormonal symptoms of perimenopause, which are an indicator that estrogen and

progesterone are not in the proper balance, taking supplements containing herbs like wild yam, black cohosh, and red clover extract may help restore balance to these two hormones and reduce perimenopause symptoms. Each of these plants is included in our Herbal Equilibrium recipe. To increase your progesterone levels, you may use a bioidentical USP progesterone cream.

These are but a few instances. Several different herbs, vitamins, and minerals may help treat hormonal imbalances. The main vitamins and herbs for

reestablishing natural hormonal balance are detailed below:
Zinc Magnesium Nutrition D
B vitamin
Iodine
Ashwagandha
Rosea Probiotic Rhodiola
Infusion of CBD

Magnesium for hormone balance.

It is appropriate to refer to magnesium as a miracle mineral given its ability to help resolve hormonal abnormalities. Your hormones may benefit from magnesium in the ways listed below: When you are under

chronic stress, your body becomes overactive. The equilibrium of the stress hormones may be disturbed by the Hypothalamic-Pituitary-Adrenal (HPA) axis. Consuming magnesium, which helps to calm the HPA and restore normal levels of the stress hormone production, you may be able to get rid of anxiety and other symptoms connected to stress. Magnesium is sometimes referred to as the "relaxation molecule" because of this.

Magnesium encourages the body's regular production of the three main sex hormones (estrogen, progesterone, and

testosterone) by aiding the liver in the metabolism of hormones and removing harmful estrogen metabolites.

Magnesium helps to rectify thyroid hormone imbalances by encouraging the conversion of inactive T4 thyroid hormones to more active T3 forms.

The magnesium's drawbacks? Most women don't get adequate support. This is partly caused by diets lacking in the mineral, but it is also because when under extreme or prolonged stress, the body "dumps" magnesium. To improve your intake of magnesium, eat more meals high in the mineral. Foods to

consume for more magnesium include spinach, black beans, edamame, cashews, and peanuts, as well as almonds, cashews, and peanuts.

Each of these foods delivers at least 15% of the daily required amount of magnesium in a single serving. Make an effort to eat as many whole foods as you can since magnesium is often eliminated during food preparation. Many women find it advantageous to take supplements to meet their 350 mg daily magnesium needs. Our magnesium citrate is designed for optimal absorption and is mild enough to be taken daily.

Additionally, magnesium citrate strengthens your heart and bones.

bitter chocolate with magnesium

For more magnesium, increase your consumption of dark chocolate! A minimum of 65% cacao content in the form of dark chocolate delivers 64 mg of magnesium per ounce. Prebiotic fiber, which feeds healthy gut flora, large levels of antioxidants, iron, copper, and manganese are all included in this delectable treat. The next time you want chocolate, try this

high-in-magnesium chocolate treat: Almonds or cashews may

be combined with little chunks of dark chocolate.

A hormone is vitamin D.

Because it is a hormonal precursor rather than a true vitamin in the traditional sense, vitamin D differs from other vitamins. The body uses vitamin D to create calcitriol, a powerful hormone that may signal more than 1,000 distinct genes to express or inhibit themselves, including genes that impact hormonal balance and endocrine function.

Vitamin D has to be met to keep the body's hormone levels balanced. Unfortunately, 42% of adult Americans lack enough vitamin D. A hormonal imbalance may be an indication that your vitamin D levels are too low. Other signs of vitamin D insufficiency include bone loss, weariness, melancholy, and cognitive fog.

How is additional vitamin D obtained?

Direct sunshine causes your skin to produce vitamin D, which you may also get via diet or supplements. Take a stroll, tend

to your garden, or just relax in your favorite patio chair for a while adopting sun protection measures, of course! Dairy and plant milk, orange juice enriched with vitamin D, various varieties of mushrooms, salmon, cod liver oil, beef liver, and sardines are among the foods that contain vitamin D. Vitamin D supplementation is a simple approach to make sure you are replacing your levels when you are aware of or think that you are lacking. A therapeutic dose of 1000 IU per

day is recommended. Look for Vitamin D3 (Cholecalciferol), which is the

most absorbable form of the vitamin, when selecting a supplement. Avoid vitamin D2 supplements and those that don't specify the kind of vitamin D they contain.

How can vitamin D assist in controlling estrogen?

Low estrogen levels have been linked to a variety of symptoms, including mood swings, migraines, sadness, hot flashes,

and more, particularly during perimenopause and menopause,

according to research. Elevating vitamin D levels aid in rebalancing estrogen.

Do omega-3 fatty acids maintain hormonal balance?

Your body needs omega-3 fatty acids, which it cannot make on its own. Therefore, you must consume them in your diet, either by eating foods like oily

fish or flaxseed or by taking supplements. In addition to being crucial for the health of your heart, bones, and brain, omega-3 fatty acids are also vital for your hormonal balance:

I. Omega-3 fatty acids increase the sensitivity of receptor sites, which are

proteins that are normally present on the surface of cells and are where hormones must "land" to transmit their chemical instructions.

II. Omega-3 fatty acids are essential hormonal precursors for the synthesis of testosterone, progesterone, and estrogen. Lack of Omega-3 fatty acids is often a contributing cause to the onset of hot flashes and other menopausal discomforts.

II. Omega-3 fatty acids are particularly good in controlling the body's out-of-control inflammation. Reduced inflammation helps the body produce hormones and protects against autoimmune conditions like

Hashimoto's thyroiditis, an autoimmune condition in which the thyroid attacks itself and may cause hormonal imbalances.

III. Omega-3s safeguard the body's capacity to produce

hormones by regulating and reducing inflammation. There is a connection between hormone imbalance and inflammation; hormone imbalance leads to inflammation, and inflammation contributes to hormone imbalance.

Hormone balance with fish oil.

Look for a high-quality fish oil that has undergone molecular distillation, a procedure that gets rid of any leftover PCBs, pesticides, solvents, and other impurities, to boost Omega-3 levels. Critical Omega-

3 fatty acids, essential fatty acids, eicosapentaenoic acid (EPA), and docosahexaenoic acid (DHA) are also concentrated in molecularly distilled fish oils. Since flaxseed oil oxidizes rapidly, it is sold in

the refrigerated part of the health food shop in dark bottles. Flaxseed oil is an excellent vegan source of Omega-3s. Because fish oils are more stable, you can be confident you're receiving the right amount of Omega-3s.

Ashwagandha for regulating hormones.

Ashwagandha helps to combat depression, stimulate libido, increase energy and focus, lower blood pressure and inflammation, and regulate

blood sugar levels as it restores hormone balance.
Recent studies on Ashwagahda as a natural remedy for PCOS, female sexual dysfunction, and reproductive issues have shown encouraging findings.

probiotics for regulating hormones.

Probiotics (healthy gut flora) are an essential component of hormone balance, which is not

surprising given how crucial gut health is for general health. Probiotics aid in reducing inflammation and enhancing

the metabolism of estrogen, progesterone, and testosterone as part of keeping a healthy gut flora, guaranteeing the balance of these important hormones. Cortisol and insulin may be brought into balance with the help of probiotics.

Where can I get additional probiotics?

Consider including probiotic-rich items in your regular diet to

increase your consumption of probiotics.

Yogurt, kefir, kimchi, fermented sauerkraut, and other fermented vegetables, and kombucha are foods that are excellent providers of probiotics. Another simple strategy to regularly replace your healthy gut flora is to take a probiotic pill. To assist in diversifying and boosting your gut health, look for a high-quality probiotic pill that contains different strains of beneficial bacteria.

B vitamins for balancing hormones.

Increasing your intake of B vitamins may assist in better hormone synthesis and balanced hormone levels throughout the body when you have a hormonal imbalance. Here are some of the B vitamins that are best for hormone health.

B12 vitamin

The liver's methylation mechanism, which breaks down extra hormones and cellular debris, requires vitamin B12 (cobalamin). Lack of B12 may prevent methylation from occurring correctly, which

might result in the accumulation

of the substance homocysteine in the blood. Increased plasma homocysteine levels are linked to hormone imbalances and may cause a variety of symptoms, including weariness, irritability, and increased inflammation.
Since animal products provide the majority of the B12 nutrient, vegetarians and vegans may be at risk for a B12 deficit. Any deficiencies in your diet may be filled with a high-quality multivitamin that includes B12.

B6 vitamin

Vitamin B6 deficiency is linked to estrogen and progesterone hormonal abnormalities. For women experiencing hormonal symptoms of perimenopause or menopause, taking a B6 supplement may be beneficial. Studies have also shown that vitamin B6 may aid with premenstrual syndrome (PMS) symptoms including mood swings and agitation. B6 should

be taken at therapeutic doses of 50 to 100 mg per day.

B3 vitamin

Niacin, often known as vitamin B3, improves liver function by

cleansing the liver of toxic substances and aids in the production of both sex and stress (adrenal) hormones. Niacin also promotes blood flow and reduces inflammation. Try to consume 16–18 mg of vitamin B3 per day.

For hormone imbalance, use CBD oil.

Cannabinoid compounds, of which CBD is one, are present in hemp and are gaining popularity for their sedative properties. Researchers didn't learn about the body's endocannabinoid system (ECS),

a network of signaling receptors that control mood, immunological responses, sleep, pain, and other functions, until decades after the 1940 discovery and extraction of CBD. Messages delivered to the nervous system, organs, and cells are influenced by the interaction of CBD and other cannabinoids with ECS receptors. Women who have hormone abnormalities due to stress may find comfort from CBD's potential effects on hormones. CBD aids in the re-regulation of the stress-activating hormone cortisol,

according to small-scale research.

Zinc for balancing hormones.

Zinc is necessary for the conversion of T4 to T3, therefore a zinc shortage may cause an imbalance in thyroid hormones and hypothyroidism symptoms. As an adaptogen, zinc helps women's estrogen, progesterone, and cortisol levels that are either low or too high. Additionally, zinc lowers inflammation, supporting the creation of healthy hormones. Meat, seafood, chickpeas and other

legumes, pumpkin, and sesame seeds are foods high in zinc.
Find a high-quality multivitamin that contains zinc in the highly absorbable form of zinc amino acid chelate to boost your levels of zinc.

Rose Rhodiola.

Cortisol control is the first step in treating an adrenal imbalance and is crucial for regaining healthy adrenal function. Your adrenal glands begin secreting cortisol, your body's primary "fight or flight" stress hormone, when your body senses that it is

under stress. Over time, the adrenal glands are tapped up by all this extra cortisol, leaving you exhausted and burnt out.

An adaptogenic plant called Rhodiola rosea (often known as "golden root") aids in rebalancing cortisol and reviving energy levels. Additionally, it improves mental clarity and supports blood sugar and the immunological system. One of the adaptogenic herbs in our Adaptisol formula for unbalanced adrenal hormones is Rhodiola.

Exercise to regulate hormones

Exercises that stimulate the body and train muscles at a more moderate intensity are the greatest for supporting hormones. Overly intense exercise may increase cortisol production, aggravating hormonal imbalances in the adrenal glands. Try these mild hormone-balancing exercises:

Walking

Going for a brisk 20 to 30-minute walk most days of the week is as easy as it gets for a cardio workout that reduces

stress, gently exercises your muscles, and increases your aerobic output. You may use a treadmill to walk indoors, but you should
attempt to get outdoors. The additional vitamin D boost from sunlight aids your body in preserving hormonal equilibrium.

Yoga

Yoga is a great way to de-stress and lower cortisol. It's also a fantastic whole-body workout for developing balance and conditioning core muscles. Having trouble with hot flashes and other menopausal signs? both swimming and water polo Try swimming and water aerobics if you often have joint pain when exercising. You can work without experiencing discomfort because of the buoyancy of the water, which relieves strain on your joints. Additionally, the additional resistance of the water increases the muscle-building power of your exercise.

Cut down on your harmful load.

Our environment now contains significantly more chemical substances. When they reach the bloodstream, several of the most widespread chemicals have estrogen-like properties that may either create or exacerbate hormonal imbalance. However, current research indicates that even modest adjustments to dietary habits and daily routines may significantly impact the environment, which is excellent news for your hormones. The following actions may be helpful:

Try easy cleaning solutions made with non-toxic components instead of harmful ones.

Limiting your exposure to chemicals and plastics may have a significant impact. We advise keeping food in glass containers, staying away from Teflon and other non-stick cookware, consuming less pre-packaged meals, and, wherever feasible, shopping for natural goods.

Your hormones need to be rebalanced immediately.

Take our hormone imbalance quiz if you suspect you may be suffering from one to better understand what your symptoms are trying to tell you.

Increase your support for your body in the first instance if your hormones are out of balance. Hormone imbalance may be treated naturally with plant-based supplements, proper diet, and lifestyle modifications. These actions taken in unison may cure the underlying issue causing your symptoms.
Our holistic approach to hormone imbalance works with

your body to gradually reestablish equilibrium.

Foods to Regulate Hormones

Hormone balance is significantly influenced by food.

There are certain meals you should aim to consume every day and others you should try to stay away from.
Healthy fats like those found in coconut oil, avocados, almonds, and wild salmon are among the foods and nutrients that support your body's ability to regulate hormones and keep you content. Magnesium is a

crucial dietary supplement, as is vitamin D. It is important to consume enough clean proteins and a lot of veggies.

Your happiness is greatly influenced by your hormones. It's crucial to keep them in check and make sure they're

operating for you correctly if you want to feel mentally well. You can regulate your hormones and have a happy, fulfilled life according to the advice given above.

Additional hormone balancing advice: Try incorporating lifestyle adjustments that promote healthy hormone

functioning as part of a natural approach to addressing hormonal imbalance. Optimal diet for hormone-balancing
Use these foods that are good for hormones to revamp your meals.

Eggs

All hormones, including progesterone and estrogen, are made with the aid of cholesterol found in eggs. Additionally, eggs contain
selenium, a mineral antioxidant that aids in removing free radicals that may harm and

prematurely age the thyroid gland.

The seaweeds.

Without iodine, your thyroid simply cannot operate. If you are insufficient, your thyroid lacks a fundamental component needed to produce enough

thyroid hormones. Women who use non-iodized
sea salt or a low-sodium diet may not be receiving enough iodine since it is added to regular table salt in the United States. Start eating more

naturally high-iodine foods like sea vegetables (kelp, duels, hijinks, noni) and seafood (clams, shrimp, haddock, oysters, salmon, sardines) to increase your intake of iodine.

Cherries

Cherry snacks may be beneficial if you have insomnia as a result of hormonal imbalances since

they are a natural source of melatonin, the "sleep hormone" produced by your pineal gland. Melatonin production declines as we age. Cherries have been shown in studies to boost melatonin levels, overall sleep duration, and sleep quality. Magnesium and Vitamin C are two additional minerals found in cherries that help regulate hormones.

Apples

A crucial substance found in apples, calcium D gluconate, aids in the liver's detoxification

of estrogen and enhances total estrogen metabolism, both of which are necessary for hormonal balance. Apple fiber aids in removing this estrogen via the intestines.

Pomegranates

The natural blocker function of pomegranates in the body helps to protect against dangerous or excessive estrogens. Anthocyanin's, which are sugarless plant pigments, and flavonoids, which are crucial for cellular detoxification and defense, are abundant in pomegranates. Pomegranates

are abundant in vitamin C, as well as vitamins A, E, and folic

acid, all of which are crucial for the formation of healthy hormones.

Flaxseeds

Lignin's, which are plant-based estrogens that support estrogen hormonal balance, are abundant in flaxseeds. Additionally, flaxseeds have healthy levels of Omega-3s, antioxidants, and insoluble fiber, which aids in the body's hormone detoxification. Add a few handfuls of flaxseeds to your smoothie or scatter seeds over a salad to benefit from this top food for hormone balance.

Avocados

Avocados are rich in beta-sit sterol, a substance that helps lower blood cholesterol and help keep cortisol levels in check. Avocados include plant sterols that affect progesterone and estrogen as well.

Nuts

Nuts, which are high in poly and monounsaturated fats, help to

maintain lower levels of insulin and cholesterol while also assisting in hormone synthesis. The following nuts promote hormonal balance:
Selenium, a mineral essential to hormone balance and support for general thyroid function, may be found in abundance in Brazil nuts.
Omega-3 fatty acids and the anti-inflammatory properties of
walnuts help to support healthy brain function.

Almonds provide wholesome protein sources and antioxidants for overall hormonal support.

Conclusion

Therefore, your life is not good. You expect better! Yes, everyone seeks happiness in life, no matter what. Happiness in life often cannot be attained by thinking about the past or the future. True happiness comes

from being content with your present circumstances and feeling good about yourself. However, as life is not always ideal, there will inevitably be ups and downs.

No matter the circumstance, you can find humor. Your approach to life's challenges will affect

how happy you are. Being happy makes you completely satisfied with life and enables you to spread pleasure to others. Simple methods of life may lead to happiness.

Make it a habit to spend some time each day thinking about

the things that make you happy. You'll feel better and more optimistic as a result of this. Many people think that chance plays a role in happiness in life and that some individuals are fated to be happy while others are.

Since happiness cannot be purchased with money, you do not need wealth or any other

kind of luxury to be happy. But how can we stop feeling stressed and depressed and genuinely start enjoying life once more? Well, there are a few simple guidelines that may improve our life. And now for them:

Know Yourself First

Recognize who you are. You must be aware of what brings you joy. Find out what gives you a sense of energy and, at the same time, what makes you joyful. Your ability to make life beautiful depends on how you act and what you do. (Stumble this)

Quit self-comparison

You could get sad if you judge yourself against other successful individuals. You must accept the fact that there will always be individuals who are more successful than you throughout most of your life. Instead, focus on others who are less fortunate and might need assistance. Your happiness level will undoubtedly increase as a result.

Participate in enjoyable activities

Although work is a necessary component of life, you may also engage in activities that bring you joy and pleasure. You can make new acquaintances, go outside, and hang around with joyful folks. You may watch a movie that cheers you up, but going to the gym or engaging in an activity is preferable.

Eat Healthy

Although eating healthy meals is preferable, you may still indulge in rich foods that might increase your pleasure. Foods like chocolates, cakes, and other

sweets may raise your mood. Your mood may improve if you go out to eat and try new food with family, friends, or both.

Go for a Break

Try pushing yourself by doing an unfamiliar task. This will increase your happiness and self-confidence. Nothing that poses a danger to society or you, of course! Go ahead and do everything you've always wanted to, such as parachute adventures, bungee leaping, or simply swimming in the ocean!

Talk it Out.

If you're depressed and need to sort things out, speak it out. Speak with someone you can trust or a member of your inner circle. You may feel better and some of the strain is lifted by just talking out your worries. You may not discover answers, but you may still feel better and be more prepared to deal with problems. Your issue could be solved if you share it.

Do something charitable

Make the time to help someone else. The experience will

undoubtedly greatly increase your happiness. Engage in charitable activity, make a donation, or volunteer at a children's charity or an elderly care facility.

Because you made someone pleased with your activities, it might make them smile and make you feel better. It offers you a reason to live, which may lead to a life of happiness and fulfillment.

Stay Concentrated

The key to success in life is maintaining concentration. Every tiny accomplishment may make you pleased and inspire you to establish new goals. You'll always look forward to tomorrow to fulfill that objective, which ultimately makes you happy.

The ultimate goal of life is to make others happy. For all of us, it is attainable. Our thoughts control our level of happiness more than our surroundings do.

As we spread our happiness in life with others, it increases our interest in helping others.

Happiness is good. Make sure you have it.

Participate in enjoyable activities

The antidotes of sadness and failure.

The antidotes of sorrow and failure.

The antidotes of sickness and poverty.

How to become smile every day

How to become smile every day

How to become smile every day

How to become smile every day

How to become smile every day

How to become smile every day

How to become smile every day

How to become smile every day

How to become smile every day

How to become smile every day

How to become smile every day

How to become smile every day

How to become smile every day

How to become smile every day

How to become smile every day

How to become smile every day

How to become smile every day

How to become smile every day

How to become smile every day

How to become smile every day

How to become smile every day

How to become smile every day

How to become smile every day

The antidotes of suffering and backwardness.